24 Energies for Advanced Healing Technology

Healing with Tachyon and Kryon Energies

Dr. Florida MAOM D.D.

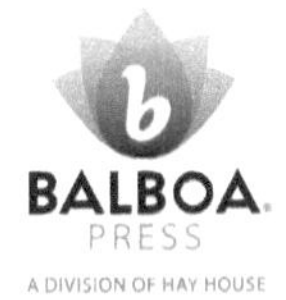

BALBOA.
PRESS

A DIVISION OF HAY HOUSE

Balboa Press books may be ordered through booksellers or by contacting:

Balboa Press
A Division of Hay House
1663 Liberty Drive
Bloomington, IN 47403
www.balboapress.com
1 (877) 407-4847

Print information available on the last page.

ISBN: 978-1-9822-1529-3 (sc)
ISBN: 978-1-9822-1528-6 (e)

Balboa Press rev. date: 05/24/2019

Dedication

I dedicate this book in loving memory of my Grandfather, who came to me in a vision during a meditative dream-state, shortly after he passed, and shared this energy technology with me.

I have been using many of the energies in my healing practice since 2012, and the effects are profound. I have received further visions, showing me that these energies would be beneficial to others for healing at a high vibration.

Contents

ACKNOWLEDGMENTS

I would like to thank all who have helped me to come to the point where I am now in my sojourn. I have had many teachers, all of whom I give great gratitude. Many of them have been authors and speakers. I have read hundreds of books and attended many healing courses and conferences on self- discovery, healing, spirituality, which have led to my specialization. I would specifically like to thank my grandfather for sharing the energies with me in a vision; Jennifer Buergermeister, who was mentor for my growth through the practice of yoga and Eastern philosophy; Dr. Bing You whom I practiced with for eight years, is my mentor in Integrated medicine, qigong and tai qi; James Tyberonn of Earth-keepers, who provided life-changing conferences that provide connections and knowledge in earth vortices and Metatronic Keys; Lois Wetzel of Hot Pink Lotus, who guided me to early important points in my journey by introducing me to higher dimensional healing modalities, Cris Jacinto who gave me the nudge to complete the book and the many other teachers I have had during my spiritual growth.

I would like to thank Christopher Morphis for his insight and beautiful art for the cover, as well as Leon Van

Kraayenburg for his sacred geometry artwork. The list could go on and on, so I would simply like to send gratitude and love to all those teachers, authors, friends, and family who have played a positive and supportive role in my journey.

Endorsements

"I have been working with these energies for several years with my patients. I am grateful for their help in balancing energy, clearing negative emotions and physical pain. The results are often instantaneous. Thank you Sara for sharing them with me."
~Erika – Houston, TX

"Sara and I became acquainted through her metaphysical group, and we were drawn closer over the years, sharing multidimensional experiences together, making us spiritual sisters. One of these amazing experiences was the birth of her son. We do meditation, energy work, and/or exchanges more consistently with our family and friends. I thoroughly enjoy Sara's work. I used to see her every week and have seen many ailments or concerns go away. It was a pleasure getting a boost and being submerged in loving clarity."
~Phire, Houston, TX

"Dr. Florida: your healing session made all the difference! Steady and daily improvement, off all meds now, and feeling very blessed as well as for the messages and insights you gave me. Thank you!!"
~T.S. M.D Family Doctor

1

∽∾

ABOUT THE ENERGIES

The 24 energies are best suited for the healers, who have experience working with energy medicine, chakras and energy balancing. These energies are advanced quantum healing technology that work inter-dimensionally and amplify energy as a compliment to other healing modalities such as Acupuncture, massage, energy work and many types of integrated healing modalities. There is a basic assumption that those reading the book have received the necessary training to prepare them for this book. There are many references available, to assist with any areas that the reader may require more study.

These energies are gifts and are to be cherished by each person who uses them. These energies are a portion of the key to the higher dimensions. The ability to use these energies opened up and became available fully to humanity in 2012 when the mass consciousness of humanity reached a vibration capable of receiving and using them on a large scale.

Basis of Tachyon and Kryon Energies

Tachyon healing energy is an energy that has been used by others on this planet for planetary and individual healing and is the basis for some of the energies in the book. The first energy we discuss will go into more detail about Tachyon energy. It is an energy that vibrates faster than the speed of light and is self- balancing. The other energies are received from higher-dimensional realms. They work within the light sphere that surrounds the earth, where human consciousness resides. "**Tachyon energy** was first defined, and its existence mathematically proven, in 1966 by MIT physicist **Dr. Gerald Feinberg**, who chose the name "**tachyon**" (from the Greek *tachys* (rapid)) because **tachyons** are subatomic particles with no mass that travel faster than the speed of light." (TerraTachyon.)

The earth resonance is ever increasing and vibrating faster as the consciousness of humanity is increasing. The earth has a heartbeat that is in alignment with the heartbeat of God. As humanity progresses and increases in vibration, our heartbeat is aligning that of Earth and God.

Several authors that have written about this energy include: David Miller of Group of Forty and Dr Joe McNamara M.D.. This book provides teachings and instruction based on the visions I received, and later added research that I found about the energies.

David Miller owner of Group of Forty, wrote "Tachyon

energy fulfills a need unmet by crystals for transmutation of life-force energy." (Miller)

According to Dr. Joseph McNamara of Tachyon Counseling, a world leader in tachyon technology information, "Tachyons are subatomic particles that travel faster than light. They are particles that infuse physical matter with spiritual light. Tachyonization is a technological process that impregnates the physical matter with an increased quantity of tachyons and thus it permanently changes quantum properties of atomic nuclei which compose that matter."

Thermodynamics plays a large role in Tachyon energy. If talking with a healer they will tell you that the energy is used for healing the body and the planet, if speaking with a scientist they will tell you it is related to energy transfer. They are both. Some physics scientists claim that this energy breaks the three laws of physics and argue that it cannot be possible. However in order to create change in this earth plane we must work faster than the speed of light. Here are the statements by a healer and a few thermodynamics physicists. Einstein says that "We can't solve problems by using the same kind of thinking we used when we created them." We can apply this principle to energy, in order to shift energy we must use a faster vibrating energy.

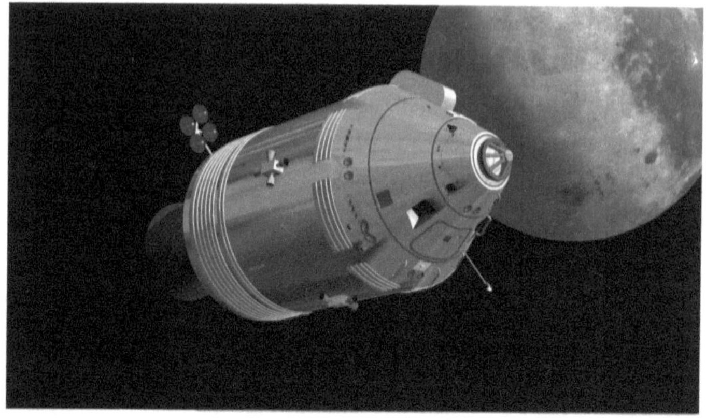

As a metaphysical practitioner I will lean toward the healing side, however I believe that they are both relevant and that this Quantum healing technology will play a large role in our future life on earth.

Kryon energies are multidimensional energies that work within the magnetic resonance of earth and are related to the vibration of the earth and the human consciousness. This energy is located in the energy sphere surrounding the globe, which allows us to work with the human consciousness and that of the earth. The balancing and changes of the energies which will be discussed in this book, work within this space. The energies themselves, when invoked, automatically work within the interdimensional aspects of earth to balance and harmonize the energies in love, light, peace, unity, prosperity, and oneness. Energies in this book that work with kryon will have the word Kryon at the end of the name of the energy.

What is Kryon? Some people who have worked with Kryon, refer to it as an angelic being that provides the means for humanity to rise in consciousness and energetic light vibration. Kryon is often channeled here on earth. The first channel was Lee Carroll in the 1980s. Quite a bit can be found about this energy through those who channel Kryon. Most of what I have received through visions and meditations is in alignment with the information I have found through verification of research. "Lee is recognized worldwide as the original channel for Kryon, and has been honored over the years by seven United Nations invitations to channel Kryon at the UN building in New York City." KRYON.COM

Lee refers to Kryon as "a loving angelic entity".

> "LOVE is the most powerful force in the entire Universe. It is the glue that will bond our belief together, instead of the doctrine that does it for the other systems. Love is not being recognized for its power, and it is not being used by us correctly."

Types of Energies: There are levels for balancing, clearing, investigating, and creating, as we will discuss in the following chapters. The first few chapters are energies that can be used daily. Each group of energies can be quite intense and may take time to master. I recommend that someone new to the energies, start by using a few energies, and mastering them before learning others. It is possible that practitioners will find five to six energies that assist them with their healing, and that is all they use. There is no need to master *all* the energies. It is best to work with the energies that call to the healer or are alignment with the work that he or she does.

Chapter 9, discusses ascension and creation energies, which are used for raising the vibration of humanity and for creation. These energies are best if used when massive global shifts are needed. Those who are guided or called to do this work, will generally already have experience and know how to integrate these energies into their work. Typically, those who do this already work in healing on a global or mass level. These energies are highly important for the overall evolution of earth and humanity. As the vibration of humanity increases, so does our ability to access these energies.

2

PREPARATION & SELF-CARE

Space Preparation

Preparing the Space: Any space may be prepared for a session for the purpose of having clean energy and protection. Space preparation can be done anywhere, and it only takes a few minutes. It is a common practice in the healing arena for highly sensitive empathic healers to prepare all spaces, prior to entering into them. It is an excellent practice to clean the energy and set the intentions of the space, prior to entering a meeting, going to a new location, or even entering your home or work on a daily basis.

How to prepare a space: Use the mind's eye, or third

eye to imagine a vortex below the space to release any "murky", lower vibrational energies from the space. Place an imaginary white dome of light over the space for protection. Imagine any lower vibrational or "murky" looking energies falling into the vortex followed by the space becoming filled with a bright light. Once the space is cleared, imagine that the vortex is closed so as to not drain your energy.

When pulling in energy, always pull it in through the crown chakra and use the universal energy rather than your own. For more information on Chakras see the self–care section.

Once the energies are learned in this book, the twenty four energies may be incorporated into the process for protecting and clearing the space. I would recommend revisiting this page frequently while learning the energies, and after completing the book to learn more advanced ways to clear a space.

Practitioner Self-Care

Daily Preparation: To be able to prepare spaces wherever and whenever needed, a practitioner is wise to keep a high level of self-care. This includes aura cleansing; energy balancing, such as tai qi, yoga, or other forms of physical health; mixed with meditation. It is recommended to do 20 minutes of self–care each morning to prepare for each day as well as regular self–care prior to healing sessions.

Using Yoga in self–care: Yoga aligns your aura with the higher dimensions up to the sixteenth. This is why people feel balanced and centered after doing yoga. To properly receive the benefits of yoga, it is best to hold each pose for one minute for the first vinyasa or set. A sensitive practitioner will feel a shift when the aura is aligned during the poses.

Daily Meditations. It is important to prepare the White Light and Align to the Sixteen Dimensions in daily meditations. As mentioned, yoga and other modalities connect to the higher dimensions, as does meditation. While doing meditation, either as a standing qigong form or as a sitting form on a chair or in lotus on the floor, the most important thing is to ensure that the feet are touching the floor and the spine is straight, to align the spine with the earth and heavens.

1. **Grounding:** First, ground yourself by imagining that you have a tree trunk in the center of your body, and the roots are going into the ground, with limbs as arms and legs. The yoga tree or mountain poses are excellent for grounding. It is best done in a green space with trees and plants.

2. **Protect** your energy by surrounding yourself and your entire energy body with a white light, calling in the energy and using the first energy called Polykryon. I will go over this in more detail when we start the energy section. This is the energy of protection. Call the energy in through your crown chakra, from the higher realms and the universe rather than using your own energy. Using your own energy for healing will exhaust you very quickly.

Two types of meditation:

1. **Mystical meditation:** a meditation in which the person sits in a quiet space, performs breathing exercises and quiets the mind. The person will allow the mind to be still and receive what comes. Remember to protect and clear prior to the meditation. People will often see images, lights, symbols, or other visions such as angles or masters. Simply allow this to occur. Many healers and lightworkers journal after meditations to record what they have received. It is common to forget what was seen after coming out of the meditation and back into the conscious mind.

2. **Manifestation meditation:** a meditation in which the person has a mantra or a desired creation through a thought form. The mantra creates instructions for the subconscious mind. For instance, the healer may say, "I am love, light, peace, unity and oneness, one with God in highest good for healing." These manifestations create the vibration of the body, the aura and the subconscious mind. This is a powerful way to change the conscious and subconscious mind rapidly. This mind programming cannot be done in a conscious state.

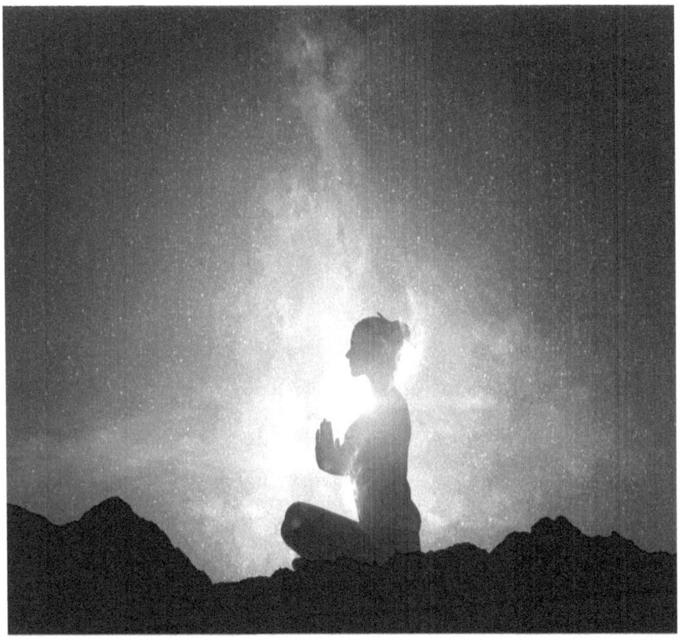

Chakra Cleansing and Preparation: Below is a brief overview of the chakra systems, for further reference, I have listed several excellent books in the reference section, that go into full detail about chakra meditations and clearing. Refer to one of these if this is not already part of your normal practice of self-healing and patient-healing practice.

The chakras have been studied by Eastern Philosophy for quite some time. The West has begun to adopt the use of them in masses more recently. Between 2001-2016, starting with the first all the way through the 16th, the chakras centers became open and available for all of humanity to access. These centers are methods to communicate with the earth, God and the universe.

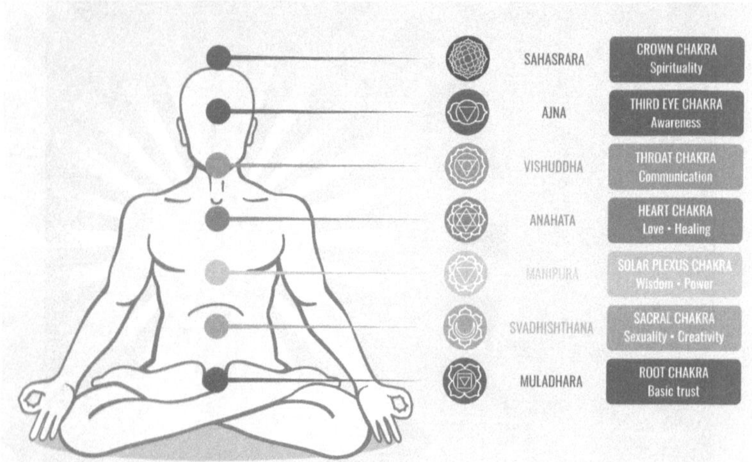

Chakra Descriptions and use:

- **Seventh, Crown:** This chakra is located on the vortex of the head. This chakra connects the person to the infinite God, and moves beyond ego and karma. Typically it is balanced in tandem with the first chakra in order to be healthy. This chakra is the location where we pull healing energies into our field from source, and may release any blockages in connecting to source. When it is out of balance or closed, a person will feel disconnected and separate from God.

- **Sixth, Third Eye:** This chakra is purple in color and is in the location of the third eye or the center of the forehead. This chakra allows us to use our abilities of foresight and intuition also known as the "mind's eye", to see that which cannot be seen with the physical eyes. We will be using this chakra throughout this book for healing and in use with the energies.

In order to use these energies properly, the third eye will require regular balancing and clarity to ensure that the information received during sessions is clear. This chakra balances spirituality and brings clarity, connects to guides, and acts as a filter for intuition and guidance. The first three chakras must be in balance and harmony for the third eye to receive clear and balanced information. I recommend that the healer be grounded and vibrating from love for clear positive reception.

- **Fifth, Communication:** This chakra is blue in color and is related to sound. When this chakra is in balance the healer or the patient will effectively use sound for healing through music, singing or language in a positive and loving way. When this chakra is opened, there is power and creativity in the spoken word. The use of this chakra can be powerful in meditations and invocations for several of the energies in this book. This chakra balances communication into love, light, harmony, and peace, and releases dysfunction in communication or even lack of communication.

- **Fourth, Heart:** This chakra is located in the center of the chest and is green in color. This chakra is related to having an open heart and in mysticism to union with universal oneness through the love vibration. The person will be aligned with the infinite light when balanced and open. Balancing this chakra will increase the vibration of love, peace, and compassion, while releasing anxiety, stress and feeling overwhelmed.

- **Solar Plexus:** This chakra is yellow in color, is located near the solar plexus where the soul is believed to reside, and also the location of the spleen. When this chakra is open and balanced it will strengthen the healing ability. This chakra balances clarity in soul purpose, divine soul alignment, willpower, and balanced divine feminine and masculine of the soul. Since this is the location of the soul it makes sense that the balance of the divine feminine and masculine will also reside here. We will talk more about this later. Those with strong second chakra perception and mind's eye may have the ability to see the soul and see when it is out of balance.

- **Second, Navel:** This chakra is located at the navel area and can be seen as a vibrant orange color. This chakra connects us with the mind's perception, astral travel, and connections to the dimensions. When first opened, there may be unclear perceptions, however, over time the clarity will improve. Emotionally, this chakra balances confidence, belief in self, ability to take action, humility, creative energy, and nurturing.

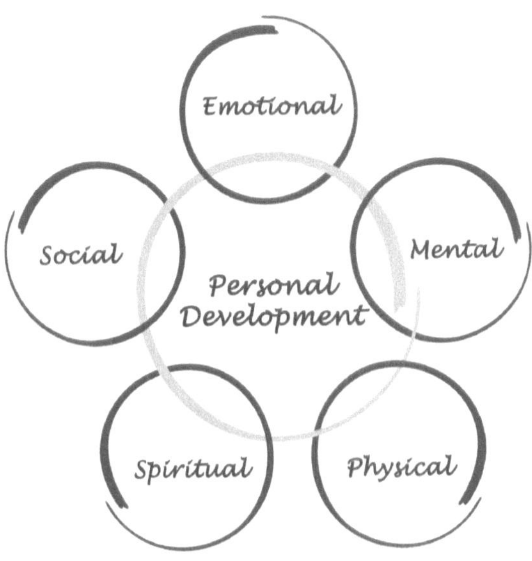

When the ego is out of balance, this chakra will also be out of balance. Often the demands on earth from a third dimensional perspective require feeding the earthly desires for power, control and superiority. These are ego based desires. The higher vibration in the fifth dimension requires more humility and less ego of power and control. The ego may be balanced in this chakra by releasing issues with power and control, and adding a more balanced healthy confidence, with trust in source.

- **First, Sacral:** This is the base chakra in the color of red, and is considered the place of awakening or the kundalini energy. When the kundalini is activated it will move up the spine and can open all of the chakras. Working with this chakra, heals issues dealing with safety, security, prosperity, sexual boundaries and faith that all is provided through source. When this chakra is not functioning properly it will be difficult for a person to function in the other chakras. Many people activate the first and other chakras through kundalini yoga.

For a deeper understanding of the chakras and how they work, please reference one of the excellent books in the reference section.

Expanding into sixteen dimensions

We often think that our aura is limited to our first 7 chakras, however in fact, once we have opened up to the fifth dimension, we have access to align with up to sixteen dimensions or chakras. Once we open up the chakra system, we are open to higher consciousness that allows us to expand our reality. In order to expand this way, first balance the first seven chakras, and open the crown chakra to align to heaven.

Steps for Expanding into the sixteen dimensions:

- Prepare the space.
- Imagine each chakra eight to sixteen being filled with a great white light.
- Use the mind's eye to determine if there are any blockages in these chakras (dimensions), imagine the white light filling it, and releasing the murky

energy into a vortex. I recommend the healer clear the energy body regularly throughout the day or weak depending on the frequency of healing work.

- Once the entire energy body is white light from chakra one to sixteen, surround it again with protection. Please see the references section for a book on the mind's eye, if more information is needed.
- Remember to close the vortex after you have completed the cleansing to conserve your energy.
- Repeat the aura cleansing of your own energy, after the session as most healers and empaths will pick up the "gunk" of those they are healing.

Other Self-Care

1. It is highly recommended to receive regular healing massages, reflexology, or acupuncture from a practitioner who understands how to balance energy and has a good positive energy that improves the practitioner's energy body.
2. Take regular baths in Epsom salts, lavender, and apple cider vinegar, as these will help pull emotional and physical toxins out of the aura.
3. Eat fresh, organic, non-GMO foods with plenty of vegetables, high in minerals and antioxidants.
4. Regular juicing and cleanses or detoxes are recommended to keep the body clear of emotional or physical toxins.

5. Get regular sleep, with naps as needed. Six to eight hours of sleep is recommended per night, to keep circadian rhythms in alignment and allow the aura to heal, as well as allowing healthy dream-state health repair.

3

PRACTITIONER ACTIVATIONS

Energy Activations: In order to be activated in using the energies, the practitioner will go through an activation process.

Self-Preparation: Prior to doing an activation, ensure to first be well practiced in the self-care.

Sit in a quiet space in a comfortable position for the meditation with the spine straight and ground the feet on the floor or sit on the floor in lotus position with the legs crossed.

- Do a full chakra clearing and balancing prior to the invocation.

- Do a full meditation prior to the invocation and maintain the meditative state during the invocation.
- Prepare a protective energy surrounding the person being activated.

Invocation: This activation need only be done once for each practitioner. It may be completed by a teacher or facilitator of the energies or oneself.

Set the following intention and say the phrases out loud.

I ____________ (say your name), hereby acknowledge that I will use the herewith in energies for the highest good of myself, humanity, the planet, and our solar system. My intentions for use of these energies are solely for healing people and the environment in which we live here on this earth. I intend to heal many people and the environment, to create a place of peace, love, unity, oneness and prosperity. I am open to receive the gift of the twenty-four energies and their inherent abilities to heal humanity and earth. I realize that the energies work through me, and I am a conduit of these energies. As a conduit, I agree to remain humble, and provide the credit for the healing, to the energies through the source of the omnipresent God. These energies will work through me, so long as I remain in a vibration of love, light, peace, unity, and oneness. I agree, that I will inform all those I directly work with, that these energies work through me as a higher technology of healing energy. I do not possess special powers as part of this healing, and the gift they receive is the gift of healing from God. I agree to obtain permission from a person prior to performing a healing on them using these energies. If the person is not open to talking about the energies, I agree to ask the person permission to perform a healing, and use my intuition or guidance to decide if the energies are an acceptable form of healing for this person. I may ask their higher self for permission as an alternative to a verbal request. Thank-you God and the higher angelic realms for bestowing upon me, this gift of healing.

SACRED GEOMETRY ACTIVATIONS

For the highest benefit of the Sacred Geometry Art, look at them in depth, and meditate with them for deeper activations within you. Sacred Geometry Art is throughout the book to add powerful activations in alignment with the energies.

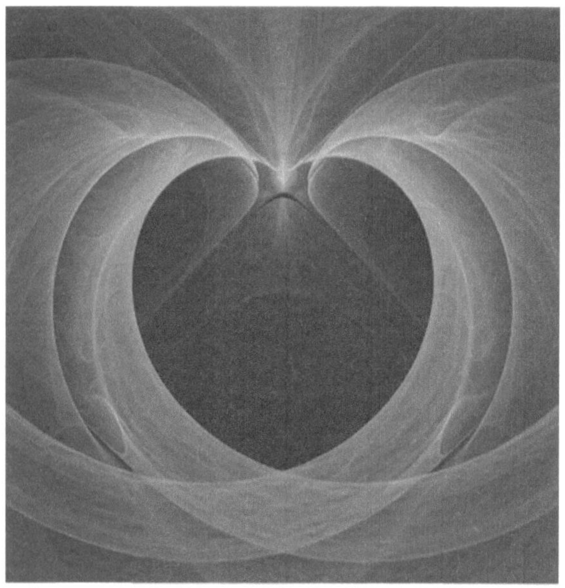

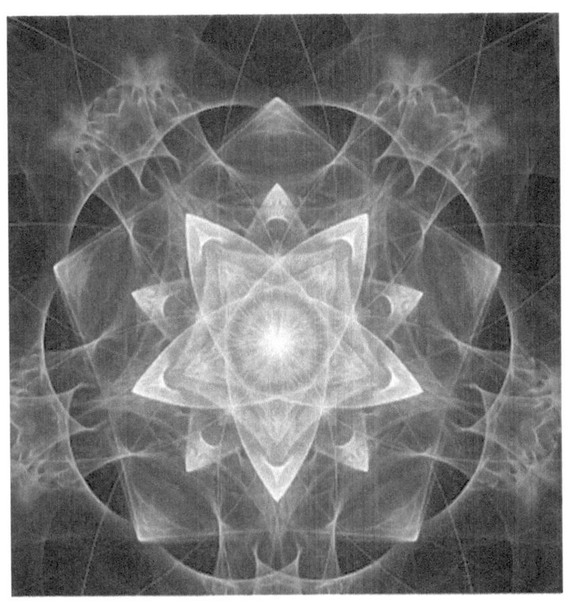

Sacred Geometry by Leon Van Kraayenburg

For the full deck of cards visit: www.sacreddnakeys.com

4

Invoking The Energies

Space Preparation:

1. Use **Polykryon** energy to create a protection around yourself and the space where the work is being done. This energy will be described in more detail in chapter 4, when we discuss the individual energies.

2. Imagine an energy vortex being placed under the space where the healing will be performed, to absorb any negative or clearing energies that will occur.

3. Enter into a meditative alpha state for invoking the energies.

4. *Generally, the space should be clean, peaceful, and have a high vibration, nice soft music, or relatively quiet, and generally feel good to the healer.* The Law of Attraction states that whatever we pay attention to, we attract.

   If there are distractions, uncomfortable loud noises, or other distractions in the healing space, these could play into the amplification of the energies.

5. If the space has any uncomfortable, "murky", or negative energies, use the clearing energies such as **Claryon** or **Negkryon** (found in the chapter on clearing energies), to clear the space prior to working on a person or performing the other work. It is an excellent practice to clear all spaces before working.

6. Once the work is complete, use the clearing energies once again to clear the space.

7. Use the mind's eye (imagination) to close the vortex under the space once complete.

Invocations for the Human Body

1. **Permission:** Obtain permission from the patient or person being healed to perform the healing process, and ask for "the highest good for the entity to be healed."

2. **Locate the Areas that Need Healing:** The practitioner will scan the space or the body that is

being healed for areas of concern using the mind's eye, intuition, and/or using hands, depending on how the practitioner sees energy. Areas of concern will often appear as murky gray or other non-vibrant colors in the mind's eye. When using the hands, the area will feel dense and heavy, depleted, or otherwise out of balance.

3. **Determine the problem:** Once the areas of concern have been determined, it is best to use intuition or guidance to understand what type of problem is at hand, so the appropriate energy or energies may be used.

4. **Set the Mode:** Say out loud or in the mind, "I work as a conduit of these healing energies from the God source in a vibration of love, light, peace, unity, and oneness to heal this person."

5. **Set the Intention:** Once the areas and type of energy needed are determined, the practitioner will set the intention of the healing session by stating out loud or in the mind what is the intention of the session, including the intended areas to be healed, and the desired outcome. When practicing, this can be written down.

    Example: "We will clear the energies that are causing anxiety and stress in this person."

6. **Direct the Energy:** The energies work very fast, so after the intention is set, the practitioner will direct

the energy to the area that is desired to heal, using the mind's eye.

7. **Invocation:** Repeat three times the name of the energy being activated while sending it to the area being healed with the mind's eye. Say the words, "I invoke this energy across all timelines, all dimensions, past, present, and future."

Invoking Multiple Energies: More than one energy may be used at a time.

For example, if an area requires physical, emotional, and past-life healing, then the three energies will all be activated simultaneously and directed at the area to be healed with the mind's eye. (Individual energies will be detailed in the following chapters with examples.) The healer would invoke: "**Tachyon, Playon, Goryon** across all timelines, all dimension, past, present and future."

Environmental Invocations: If the energy is being invoked to heal something in the environment, such a green space or pollution, there are a few changes to the protocol. Instead of directing the energy toward a person, it will be directed in a dome shape to the area being healed. The invocation is the same.

Permission: Obtain permission from a higher self or ask that the energies be used in the "highest good for all involved."

Time: In the higher dimensions, time does not exist as it does in the third dimension in a linear fashion. When energies are invoked, sometimes results can occur immediately, and other times, they may take time. When I say *time* in linear, third-dimensional time, it could be days, weeks, months, or even years. Most of the time, there will be some indication that a plan is taking shape and changes are beginning to occur. Each energy is different in how it manifests.

For example, when using Tachyon, the energy for physical ailments, it could begin to manifest in that the person receives a strong pain in the digestive system that requires him or her to research the ailment further, by reading or even obtaining some testing for the digestive system. This could lead the person to realize that taking a certain vitamin or mineral will correct the digestive dysfunction.

Sometimes the energies will work and make great changes on their own, and other times the energies will guide the person to a series of events that will cause the healing to occur. I have used this thousands of times for myself and for patients.

For example, I once had a skin condition that I tried many ways to remedy, and it was not healing to my satisfaction. Once I used the energies, I was led through a series of events to determine the healing protocol. The energies help to automatically balance any imbalance that may lead to a condition, and assist with the immediate surroundings to bring what is to be healed into balance. It can manifest in many ways and in multiple timelines and throughout all dimensions, past, present, and future.

In the fifth dimension and higher, all of time exists at one point in the present moment. This is difficult to grasp from a third-dimensional, linear point of view; however, it is the case. When the energies are activated, they can heal the issue in all of time. For example, in the movie, *Back to the Future*, when an action changed, it affected the future. This works the same way. If, when activated, the energy heals a situation from the past, it will affect the current situation as well as the future.

Examples: When invoking the energy for creating green space, **Pimikryon**, whether this person is planning to do gardening or not, the energy will invoke the energy to create a green space. Sally may invoke this energy in a place that has no green, and she may find that the city initiates plans to create a new green space in the location where she invoked the energy. A second example: perhaps a neighbor fails to take care of his yard, leaving the street looking less than desirable. If the energy is invoked on that yard, it will be amazing to see that within higher-dimensional time and reality, that yard will be transformed. Perhaps you will see the neighbor suddenly takes initiative to care for his yard, or he hires a landscaper. The energy works in ways that are not easily understood by the third-dimensional linear mind. I have witnessed this many times. Living in Houston, I frequently drive down polluted and unkempt streets. (Many streets are beautiful and full of trees.) When I travel on these streets, I will often invoke the energies, and I am always pleased by the eventual transformation of these areas. I have done the same on my own street, which is an older street with houses built in the 1960s. Since I have invoked the energies on my street, six houses on the street have been remodeled and made to have much higher vibration and beauty.

Intent: When working with the energies, it is best to set a positive intention of the outcome that you would like to occur.

Manifestation and Allowing: It is best to invoke the energies with an intention of allowing. Our mind-set will influence the outcome, a positive mind-set with full trust that our manifestation will occur, will bring about the highest and good. We invoke the energy, create our manifestation, allow and trust. We allow with confidence, with patience, and from a place of peace. If we are working on patients, it is wise to train them to "allow" the healing to occur as it does. Give them the expectation that all will occur in the divine timing, on a nonlinear scale. Anxiety, stress, and impatience will block the energies and the manifestations. Again, remember: *manifest our creations in peace, and allow in patience.*

Patient State of Consciousness: Generally, it is necessary to use these energies on healing subjects who are open and receptive to energy healing. I have experimentally used the energies on people that are not overly receptive to them, and I have found that they client may sometimes have an emotional backlash response such as anger or resentment. They must be open, appreciative and receptive for the energies to work properly. This will require a level of intuition and knowing from the healing practitioner. If you are unsure about this, I highly recommend studying the characteristics of the fifth dimensional consciousness further before proceeding with the energies. Many books are listed in the references section at the end of this book.

When the consciousness is in the higher dimensions, the energies are more likely to work on the patient. I have been guided to focus these energies on these higher-vibrating patients for the sheer reason that their energy bodies will be compatible with the energies. This requirement is only the case with humans. If they are not ready for this level of healing, it could be a shock to the system. It would be like bringing in HD television to a tube television. Objects and spaces are capable of receiving the energies.

5

Physical And Emotional Healing Energies

These energies are the basis for the twenty-four energies and are used most frequently. They are used to heal emotions and physical space that are directly observable in our current situation, spaces around us or patients. They can all be used by themselves, or in combination with any other energy in this book. I highly recommend learning the energies in this chapter first, and becoming comfortable with them prior to learning the other energies.

Guided versus Automatic Healing

Automatic: Each of the energies are capable of healing, using the invocation process with little or no guidance from the practitioner other than setting the intention of the energy and allowing. The healer may choose the energies needed for the healing and invoke multiple energies at one time.

Guided: Use the mind's eye to see or feel energies, and guide the energy appropriately. The healer will be more actively involved in the healing session, and have more insight as to what further energies need to be invoked for the healing. If the person being healed is open to it, the healer may share what is occurring.

1. **POLYKRYON**

Protection: This energy is the most important in the twenty-four energies and is to be invoked every time any of the energies are used. It is used as protection while doing work and throughout the day. It appears as a shimmering platinum yet clear color. This energy is the one to be used during preparation and anytime practitioners feel they need to protect their energy. The purpose of the protection is to provide a shield from any forces that may reside in the surrounding space, timelines, or dimensions that are not in the highest good of the work. It is important to invoke this energy in a feeling of love, light, safety, and security. If there are any fearful feelings, it is best to avoid using the energies.

Use: During invocation, imagine that the platinum shimmering energy is surrounding the practitioner's energy body as well as the energy body of the person or the area to be healed. This can be done multiple times in a session or throughout the day as needed. Review the invocation process for the full invocation of this energy in conjunction with the other energies.

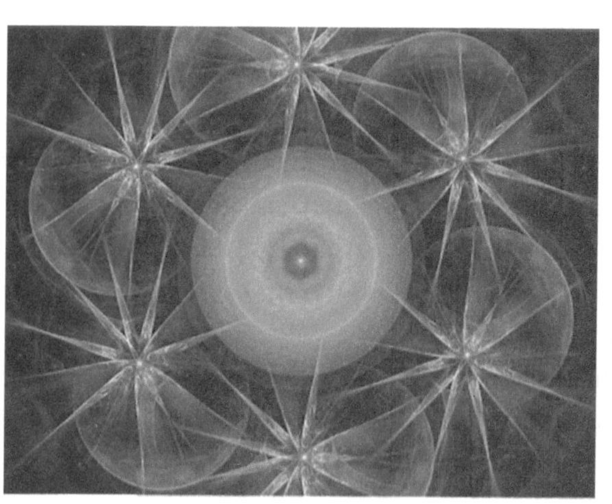

2. TACHYON

Physical ailments: this energy balances physical manifestations and is already well known on earth. It is an energy that is like a white shimmering platinum color that vibrates faster than the speed of light. The purpose of this energy is to clear physical health ailments and pain. It does so by creating a vibration faster than the physical pain or ailment and transmuting it back into health.

Use: Follow the invocation we have learned previously and focus attention on the area of the body that is inflicted with poor physical health or pain. Imagine this platinum shimmering energy engulfing this space. This energy, like the others, will balance and begin the healing process automatically; there is no need to do additional balancing work for this area of the physical body. It can be used in conjunction with other healing modalities such as acupuncture, massage, herbs, oils, etc. It is not recommended to combine this with other forms of energy works outside of the twenty four energies, (such as reiki), as it stands alone. It is best to do the other forms of healing first and then apply the Tachyon energy to complete the process.

Healing from Tachyon energy, like the others, is automatic and may come in many forms. It may lead a person to seek out a new kind of healing they had not thought of before, it may assist the individual with guidance for the perfect remedy, or it may heal the person at that time. These occurrences could be through divine intervention, such as a friend suddenly talking about it or a stranger telling the person about an herbal remedy. As we discussed, allow time to manifest in the divine fifth-dimensional nonlinear time. The person will usually feel relief and may report experiencing interesting and unexpected healing. Tachyon will provide or guide a person to the highest healing for his or her condition.

Healing Etiquette: Do not interfere with this process by giving excessive advice to the person beyond providing the healing during the initial session. It is beneficial to the process to check in with the person about his or her healing regularly and ask about progress. Allow for the energies to work and guide you and the patient to what steps will be next. You may hear some interesting and profound stories. Tachyon may be used multiple times until the healing is complete, but be sure to allow it to do its work. Overuse and anxiety about the outcome could block the energies.

If individuals are not open to the use of the energy, they are not of the vibration to use it, so it is best not to use it on them. There are many other subtler healing modalities available for this case. I have used this energy most commonly with the most outstanding results. This energy has been received and used by others on this planet, so this book is not the first introduction. I have reviewed their work, after using it for quite some time, and it has given validation to me, about the use of the energies.

3. PLAYON

Playon is the energy that balances the emotional body. This energy looks like a thin, ray of thin and nearly transparent crystalline light in multiple colors according to the chakra colors.

Use: The best use of it is to identify the emotions that need to be released and focus this energy to the part of the body or the part of the earth where these emotions are residing. Use the mind's eye to see the energy of the area to be healed and determine the color of the emotion to be released. The color chart is listed below.

Invocation: Repeat the word *Playon* three times and allow. This energy is automatic and will create release and balancing on its own, so there is no need to focus on the healing for an extended time. Invoke the energy, and allow it to do its work.

This energy is automatic. However, if a specific area of the body or the aura is being worked on or a certain emotion, the following colors may be guided to the area for clearing or reinforcing by imagining the area being filled with the appropriate color. Release the non-vibrant or murky colors and direct the new vibrantly colored energy to the area.

Aura/Chakra Colors: Negative and Positive:

- White: Clears sadness, depression, disconnectedness from spirit and source
- Purple: Clears clutter and blockages to spirituality and intuition

- Blue: Clears blockages in communication or negativity in communication
- Green: Clears anger, disgust, judgment, anxiety, and indecision of the heart, issues of not feeling connected, and lack of love
- Yellow: Clears worry, confusion, and self-doubt, lack of direction, issues related to self-will and disharmony between masculine and feminine
- Orange: Clears negative excessive ego triggers, inaction, laziness, issues with confidence, creative blockages, and infertility
- Red: Clears lack and fear, insecurity, issues related to being grounded, and safety-related issues

Use the chakra system to rebalance the emotions. Begin with the first chakra, to rotate the chakra counterclockwise and release all that no longer serves, and do this for each. Activate the energy on each chakra while they are open. Imagine the energy flowing out of each until you see that all the negative vibration energies have been released. The energy will automatically release the negative and replace the positive.

For those not familiar with the chakra system, this is only a brief overview, I recommend studying this further prior to using the energies. I have provided a brief overview of the chakra system in the self- care chapter of this book as well as a few excellent books on advanced chakra healing in the reference section of this book.

6

CLEARING ENERGIES

The purpose of these energies is to clear out what no longer serves us. These can be used in people, objects, or spaces.

4. **CLARYON**

Clarity and release of clutter: This energy is best used when we have a cluttered mind or space. It is beneficial when we notice that we are receiving multiple mixed messages, manifestation is not as fast or clear as usual, our intuition is unclear, we have a hard time making decisions, we feel overwhelmed, or feel ill at ease with our surroundings because of too much clutter.

Use: To invoke this energy, follow the invocation steps; identify which areas of life, mind, or space need clearing or clarity, and call out the name three times, saying *Claryon*; then allow it to manifest. This is an automatic energy requiring no further action.

Manifestation: Results can range from immediate to several weeks. You will feel a shift and receive spiritual and intuitive guidance on what needs clearing. You may ask, *If I have no clarity, how will I receive the guidance?* The answer is that the energy will assist in making this information clear for you. This can range from intuitive guidance, having a desire releasing objects from your home or work space, releasing tasks or thoughts that are cluttering your mind, or even a recommendation for healing your physical, spiritual or mental bodies. An example may be a detox protocol or eliminating a certain food from your diet.

It is best to do a daily five-minute meditation with journaling to receive the messages necessary to carry out the actions. The energy may balance some of your thoughts and energies for you automatically. It may be necessary for you to do some balancing yourself during your meditations and using the chakras, so you may be aware of the healing process and change related thoughts, feelings, habits or behaviors that are no longer serving you.

5. **NEGKRYON**

Release negativity: This energy is used to release negativity from the human and earth energy bodies. Imagine it as a vacuum that is sucking out negative gray or murky energies. It can be used on a person's energy body or any space on earth. When it is determined that negative energies are present, follow the space preparation and invocation process. Invoke Negkryon energy and direct it toward the negativity that you wish to be released. The negativity can be a thought, a belief, a situation, or a space.

Use: Imagine the "murky" energies being sucked up through a vacuum hose into the vortex that was created. This energy is automatic like the others and need only be invoked with intention and then allow it to do its work. Once the session is complete and the mind's eye sees that the "murky" energies are cleansed into light, and the vortex may be closed.

This energy is often used in conjunction with **Playon Energy** to balance the emotions. Negkryon will release the negativity, and Playon will balance them.

Patient Care: The energy will continue to work after the session is complete, so it is good to advise the patient to take a nice bath in Epson salts or apple cider vinegar to assist with the release, and be aware that his or her emotions may feel strong for a few days while they are clearing. The patient can be advised to get extra rest and inform family members and friends that he or she is doing emotional work and that strong emotions may suddenly arise. The patient could journal and keep in touch via e-mail or phone, to let the practitioner know how the patient is feeling.

6. ANKRYON—(Ankh)

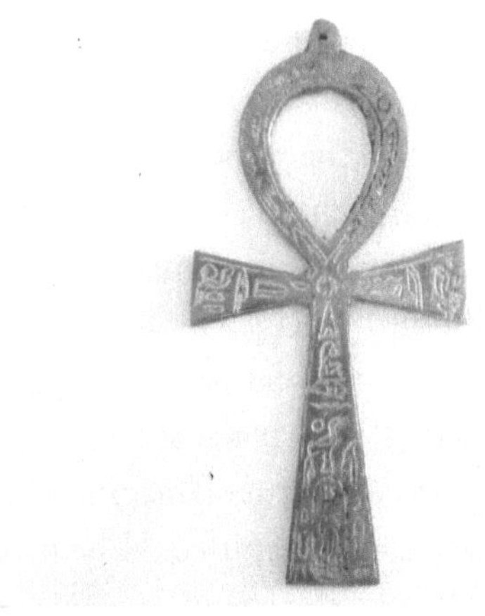

Clear imbalances in feminine and masculine: This ancient symbol of life and fertility represents the balance of the male and female. The Egyptian cross is a powerful energetic tool for eternal life. The ankh symbol can be used energetically to balance the divine feminine and divine masculine through clearing imbalances and unification. This harmonization into perfect union is essential to raising the vibration and eternal life of the soul.

Use: This energy is most appropriate when an energy body needs balancing of the divine feminine and masculine to equality. The use of this energy will increase the vibration of the energy body and open the energy body up to rapid growth and expansion.

To use the Ankryon energy, imagine the ankh over the chakra being worked on, and follow the invocation process. Use the mind's eye to place this symbol on the energy body, and it will perform the work of the energy. It may be placed on one chakra or all sixteen.

7. PIMIKRYON

Clearing, balancing, and healing green spaces: This energy can be used in a space of any size. It is best to use it in a space that is easy to see in the mind's eye or imagination.

Examples: These may include a garden in the backyard, healing a forest, or maybe even an area that lacks green space and needs it in the middle of a city.

Use: Set the intention of what is to occur in the area, imagine the space as it is, and place an imaginary white platinum energy dome over the space. Imagine it converting into the beautiful green space that it could be by using the invocation process to invoke the energy.

How it works: This energy does not require the practitioner to perform anything physical. The practitioner does not need to hire a team of landscapers and develop a budget to make this work. The energy will occur on its own.

Example: say I were to invoke the energy in a downtown area over a space that is desired to heal, clear or balance. I later return to the space, perhaps weeks or months later. A local developer has decided to remodel a building and add a small park to the area. If I did this at my home and lacked the time to do it myself, within a period of time, perhaps my neighbor would come over and offer to weed my yard and plant new plants free of charge if I provide plants. (That is a true story.)

Time: Like the other timeframes we talked about, the time will be according to the universal plan. When you do the invocation, ask that it be done according to the divine plan, and it will. This could be days, weeks, months, or years in linear, 3-D time. The important part is to invoke and allow. Check back to see the progress.

7

INVESTIGATIVE ENERGIES

These energies are best used for investigation, researching, or finding out answers related to the necessary healing. This is a more advanced form of healing for the seasoned healer. These energies are useful in healing a person, place or thing, when we must first determine why it is out of balance in the first place. These energies can be used for cases that are less obvious and require deeper understanding for the healing to occur.

For example, if someone came to a healer for healing of a pain and had an obvious injury, this would have a cause and no need for deeper answers. However, if a person came to the healer and had a lifetime of pain in an area of the body that had no explanation, no doctor could find any reason for the pain, this would be a reason to do further investigation to determine the underlying cause. Typically, this energy is useful if the energies for balancing and clearing have not completely healed the issues at hand. Healers who use these energies typically have a form of connection with the divine, in which they are able to receive information from the subconscious of the earth plane, humanity, multidimensionally, or across all timelines.

Methods to Receive Answers Using These Energies

Automatic: The energy is invoked, and it clears on its own without the information entering into the conscious mind of the healer or the patient. Neither will be aware of what occurred or healed. However, in the multidimensional divine timeline, changes and healing will occur.

Guided: The practitioner may access this information for the person or guide him or her to receive the information by going into a meditative state. This option will be based on the capabilities of the healer and the willingness or openness of the patient. Both the healer and the patient will become aware of the incidents that occurred and will be healed. The healer will say aloud or write through automatic writing, the information that is received during the session. It is a common practice to use a voice recording for the session and provide it to the patient.

Guided Method 1: Automatic Writing will require going into a meditative or alpha state to receive the information. The healer and the person being worked on can use breathing exercises to reach this state. If the person being worked on is comfortable doing so, he or she can perform the automatic writing. If the person is not comfortable doing the automatic writing, the healer may do the automatic writing for him or her. I only recommend this for healers who have experience doing this type of work. This takes practice and study on the part of the healer.

How automatic writing works: Have a pen in hand with blank paper while going into the meditative state. It is best to use a book or multiple sheets of paper, so as to not break the flow state during the process. The healer will receive the information and allow it to flow through the pen without thinking about what is being said. They will write whatever comes into their mind. The writing could occur over one session or multiple sessions if needed. Oftentimes the handwriting will not be the same as the person's normal handwriting, and it could even be difficult to decipher. Once it is clear that the session is complete and no more information is coming, the healer and patient can read the information to determine how it can assist in the healing process.

Guided Method 2: Imagery through Meditation, occurs when the healer goes into a meditative alpha state and guides the patient. There are many ways to do this, so I recommend the practitioner use the method he or she is most comfortable with. The healer can receive images for the person and say them out loud or write them or, if capable, the patient may allow images to flow into her mind's eye while in the meditative state, so that she will see the answers that are requested.

Sharing: It is not necessary for the practitioner to share everything that comes up in the session, if it would make the patient feel uncomfortable. There may be instances when the information that comes up is so traumatic or painful that it is best to simply clear it rather than invoke the energy into the conscious mind of the person being healed. If the person being healed is not completely open to the information that will come up, it is best to use the automatic form and allow it to heal on its own. As long as the person has given permission for healing, the healing can be performed.

Timing: The answers may come at different times however, unlike the other energies, these energies tend to be more instantaneous. Often the answers will come immediately while in a meditative state. If they do not, the person will continue to go into regular meditative states until the answers come to them. The reason this is instantaneous is because the answers already exist in the multidimensional level and only need to be received. Timing is based more on the receptive ability of the healer or person seeking the answers.

8. **LORYON**

Lost Language or Words: This energy is most beneficial when someone is lacking the words for what he or she is trying to say. Often people will say something like, "I have lost the words" or "there are no words to describe it." These thoughts are frequently at a multidimensional level, and the person is unable to access the words or the language because the thought is residing at a different level of consciousness than the spoken third-dimensional language.

Use: Invoke this energy using the regular process, then ask the person to set the intention of the words that he or she wishes to retrieve. Use one of the reception methods above to retrieve the lost words. This energy is directly related to the fifth chakra of communication and sound. Sound healing using Tibetan or crystal bowls, drumming, singing, chanting, invocations or other sound healing are encouraged to be used with this energy. This energy is self-balancing and will work on its own.

Example: A patient had a severe sinus infection, which entered the brain and required brain surgery by a surgeon. The patient had lost use of half of his body and his speech. After his surgery his mobility returned, however his speech did not. During the recovery phases with physical therapy, we activated the Loryon energy to re-activate his speech. Between the physical treatments he was receiving and the energy healing, he was able to regain his speech.

9. **FORKRYON**

Making Decisions: As the name indicates, this energy is most useful when there is a decision or a "fork in the road." The patient is seeking answers to decisions.

Use: There are multiple steps to using this energy. First, write down the possible outcomes of the decisions, and use the third-dimensional decision making strategies such as a comparison of pros and cons, prior to invoking the energy. Once the analysis is complete, both the healer and the subject will go into the meditative state, and use the invocation process to set the intention of the information that is desired.

For retrieval of answers, use either the "**visionary meditation**" method to view the possible outcomes of the decision or the "automatic writing" method, to write down the potential outcomes. Finally, when receiving the outcomes, place one hand on the heart and feel how the decision feels in the heart. The decision is best made, based on the compilation of the received information, the analysis and the feeling in the heart. The right decision will "feel right", and be clear. Repeat the process until the decision is clear.

Negative emotions related to decisions: When a decision brings up any feelings of negativity, funny feelings, hesitation, anxiety, or upset in the gut, pay attention and ask for clarification to these feelings. The feelings may need clearing, and it would be best to explore them further by using the energies for balancing and clearing, prior to making the decision. When a decision brings up these feelings, it does not necessarily mean it is completely wrong.

It may mean the person has a blockage or area that needs healing prior to making the decision.

Example: A person is debating if she should visit her long-lost parents, that would require her travel by airplane. The parents have written a long letter talking about how much they would love to see her. We know that there will be a positive reception on the other hand. While going through the decision process, it is determined that she has an anxiety about traveling on a plane, which stems from the loss of a family member on an airplane at an early age. The feeling has nothing to do with seeing the parents. Once the true cause of the feeling is determined, this fear can be eliminated, so the real decision can be made. Now we ask the question again, "Should she go visit her long-lost parents?" In the process, anxiety may also come up about seeing them for the first time. All the negative emotions would be addressed prior to making the decision. Once the fear of airplanes is addressed and anxieties about seeing the parents are cleared, the person is able to make a decision based on what her heart wants. After looking deeply, receiving some answers and feeling her heart, she decides that she would love to meet them. She may find that her heart yearns to meet her parents, and she is willing to overcome the obstacles in order to do that.

A good decision will feel good, positive, energetic and enthusiastic, with a mood of being ready for action. Repeat the clearing process until the answer feels this way.

10. **SLEPLYON**

Dream State: During the dream state, we create, we learn, we travel to many places, we heal, and we regenerate. Invoke this energy before falling asleep, for best results, when important answers, healing, or mental cleansing is needed. We often process our subconscious mind in our dreams.

Use: Use the invocation process before falling asleep, and go into a meditative state when falling asleep. It is important to invoke the protection before all the energies are used; however, it is especially important before using the dream-state energy. During sleep, we are unable to protect ourselves consciously. This will ensure that no entities or unwanted energies interrupt the process.

Caution: Refrain from using this energy when the mind is less than positive as negativity such as anxiety, fear or stress will have a negative result on the dream state. It is wise to place a bowl of Himalayan salts in a bowl under the bed to absorb any negativity during this process and be sure to create the vortex for clearing.

Recording: When awakening, have a journal nearby to write down any and all that you remember from the session and journal any changes that occur during the following weeks because of the session. It is recommended that the sessions be invoked on average once per week, with a maximum of three times, if there is a time when quite a bit of trauma or negativity is coming up that needs clearing.

11. **GORYON**

Past Lives: This energy is best used when it is determined that a person is afflicted by incidents from a past life that are affecting his or her present life, emotionally, physically, spiritually, or intellectually.

Use: Choose either guided or automatic retrieval.

Invocation: Use the standard invocation process and retrieval methods. If using the automatic method, this is all that is required. For a guided retrieval, follow the process and once the past life is revealed or the incidents leading up to the blockage are seen, release the past life trauma and incidents that no longer serve the patient.

Releasing: Imagine the traumas or incidents of the past life as a gray, dirty energy sinking into the vortex. Imagine the person or human consciousness being whole and healed in the area that was affected by the past life. Fill them with a vibrant white light that fills any areas that were released. When setting the intention, set both the trauma that is to be healed as well as the intended outcome. Finally, close the vortex and allow the energy to complete any additional work that is needed.

Example: a person is having a financial difficulty, he consistently receives his paycheck and spends it all quickly, leaving him with no money and large amounts of debt from using credit cards. After carefully looking at his life patterns, he has determined that nothing has occurred in his present life, such as childhood beliefs, that could lead to this behavior, so he seeks to find out what is causing it. While doing the session, the practitioner through "visionary meditation", determines that there may be a past-life incident involved. They can now move forward with the healing. After the healing and in divine timing, the patient may become more sensible with money and set aside a certain percentage of it, without frustration or anxiety. He may also find that a series of events occurs that forces him to become better with his money.

Automatic versus guided session: It is not necessary to retrieve the past life trauma, if it is determined the trauma is based on a past life, simply invoke the energy and allow it to heal the past life. If preferred, you may use the guided method, which allows more insight to the patient from an analytical point conscious of view, but it is not necessary to perform the healing.

12. **GNOSKRYON**

Access the book of knowledge: Investigate for karma, phobias, fears, and anxieties in all timelines and all dimensions. Use this energy in combination with **Goryon,** as there is often a tie to past lives. This is helpful when a person is having a blockage to expanding or shifting. It can be valuable when the patient feels stuck or is having anxiety about a situation in life. The patient may have a belief that was ingrained into the subconscious, which is blocking him.

Use: The practitioner and patient will go into a meditative state and use one of the methods for retrieval. The invocation of the energy may clear the blockages using the automatic or the guided methods of retrieval.

Retrieval Method: The automatic method is much faster, and may be the preferred method for this energy, as using the guided method would bringing the thought to the conscious mind and manifest issues into the current life, whereas the automatic method will release the trauma without affecting the conscious mind.

Invocation: Set the invocation with the focus on the fear, anxiety, or situation that is to be cleared, and ask "that the highest good occur to clear this situation."

8

VIBRATION RAISING ENERGIES

Energies in this chapter are used to raise the vibration of a person, place, or community. As a collective, humanity has made many shifts in vibration over the past few hundred years. Over the past 100 years and especially since the year 2000, the speed at which our vibration is increasing is phenomenal. Similar to the way our technology is always updated and becomes obsolete, the human vibration is constantly shifting upward.

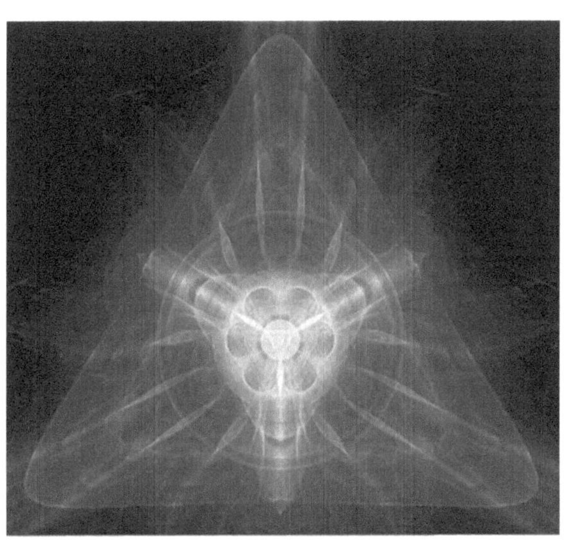

13. **COLKRYON**

Collective Conscious: This is the energy of healing the collective conscious. There are many reasons to use this. Over time, humanity has created many things. Some creations have served us well, and others have created problems on earth that are not in our highest good. These energies will clear any mis-creations we have created here on earth that no longer serve us.

Use: To use this energy, set the intent of connecting human consciousness with that of the vibrations of the higher dimensions. In order to do this, the practitioner must be aligned and in tune with these higher dimensions. This energy, as with the others, will only work when it is invoked from a vibration of love.

To set the intention, first determine the conscious thoughts that are prevalent in society that no longer serve the collective conscious and invoke the Colkryon energy. Once the conscious thoughts that are desired to be released or transmuted are determined, then imagine the consciousness that will take its place, and ask the Colkryon to transform the conscious in the higher good of humanity and to raise humanity into the fifth dimension.

Example Invocation "Release the collective conscious energy of fear that is prevalent in our society today into one of peace and higher vibration of love." Imagine, if masses of humanity used this energy daily to heal our planet, the rapid changes that would occur.

14. **PISTEUYON**

Earth Heartbeat: The earth heartbeat is tuned to the universal heartbeat of God. When humanity is aligned with higher vibrations and in harmony with the earth heartbeat, humanity is at peace. The activation of this energy will align the person, group, or community with the earth and God heartbeat of peace, unity, love, oneness, and prosperity.

Use: This energy can be used to heal situations when the patient is feeling overly stressed, anxious overwhelmed and generally out of alignment with the earth balance. This energy is highly effective when doing work with the fourth heart chakra as it relates directly to the heart and love vibration, which aligns with the heartbeat of the earth.

Example: when humanity becomes to preoccupied with power and ego we can become mis-aligned with the universal oneness, which aligns with the heartbeat of earth. If one had found that they were not feeling grounded and had excessive anxiety, this could indicate that their aura is fractured and they are not aligned with the earth energies. Activating this energy will calm their aura and the anxiety as well as align them with the natural flow of the earth energy and universal oneness.

15. SANGYON

Sound Healing: Known as the song of light. This energy is used to heal sounds and raise the vibration of the sounds, so they may be amplified into light. Examples of the need for sound healing would be ailments, emotions, or situations that bring discordance to the ears or hearing.

Use: Many healers use sound healing to work with the vibration of spaces and the energy of the body for healing. Gongs, crystal bowls, and music of all types can be used for healing and balancing the energy body. When used properly, sound and music are extremely healing. When improper sounds are used, they can disrupt the energy flow in the body, a space, or the earth frequencies. There are frequencies that bring about healing, which can be studied further by those interested in this area. This energy will balance, heal, and amplify the sound frequencies of a person, space, area, or even the planet.

When using this energy, it is ideal to have a high-frequency sound from either a gong or a Tibetan or crystal bowl to assist with the healing. It is important to invoke the energy when the sounds in the presence of the invocation are of a high frequency with little or no other sound around. This energy primarily works with the fifth chakra of communication and is ideal for balancing this chakra.

Example: Invoking this energy on a noisy freeway or at an airport near planes taking off, would project that sound energy and increase it, so it is best to use this one during a meditative state in the presence of a beautiful high-frequency sound. It can be used to balance noisy areas or sounds, even from a distance. For instance, if there were an unpleasantly noisy area near a patient's home, perform the invocation in a private and pleasant-sounding area, and set the intention to project the pleasant sound into the area with the unpleasant sound.

Space Preparation: Many of the other energies could be invoked in many spaces, however, this energy is important to invoke in a quiet place where the sound is controlled. The preparation is highly important, as whatever occurs in the space related to sound, can be amplified into the healing.

Intention and Clearing: The order of intention is important for this energy. If there are discordant energies or sounds to be cleared, first clear the space using the clearing energies discussed in the earlier chapters. Direct these clearing energies at the area to be healed. After clearing the sounds, set the intention of the energy or sound that the healer would like to amplify. Sound and instruments are the best method for setting the intention using—gong, bowl, music, singing, humming, or whistling. If silence is desired, use complete silence.

Example: There are times when all of us need assistance from our fellow healers. I have a few of my favorite spiritual healers that I go to when I need extra alignment. I enjoy going to crystal bowl sound baths and meditations. One of my favorite healers named Harry uses gongs and bowls surrounding a healing table. He is guided by intuition as to what to play to help release and balance the energy body. Love these sessions and find that they can balance emotions, vibrations and even traumas that are not balanced in other methods. I have done this type of healing when there are huge world events or great trauma with my patients and as an empath, I have received an overload of stimulus. I reiterate here the importance of clearing and protection regularly as an empathic healer.

16. **SALVYON**

Infinity Energy: This energy implies salvation into the infinite eternity, which is essentially the goal of many people on earth. This involves raising ourselves and our planet to a higher vibration that is sustainable for eternity. Our light bodies and our planet will continue to rise to higher dimensions and frequencies. We will not disappear into thin air; it simply means we are upgraded to a higher vibration. Humanity is awakening now in masses of millions per month. There are thousands who have anchored the light for hundreds of years. 144,000 lightworkers have heralded in this time of increased vibration for humanity. We are now at a time of critical mass, when the masses are waking up and moving into the higher vibrations of love, light, peace, unity, prosperity, and oneness.

Humanity have evolved on earth in outstanding leaps in only one hundred years. This is a quickening and an opportunity to ascend into the fifth dimension and beyond. Many of us are already vibrating in these higher-dimensional frequencies, and many more are rapidly approaching. The purpose of this energy is to assist all of humanity in this process.

When invoked, this energy will raise the vibration and consciousness of humanity incrementally. This incremental increase in vibration and consciousness of humanity has been occurring for quite some time on earth. The increases in vibration for humanity have been accelerating as time approaches closer to the year 2034 which is considered the completion of the ascension. Activations began in 2000 which created shifts up and each year we have had new energy up shits with major ones occurring in 2012. It is now quickening at a pace so rapid that the daily changes are astounding.

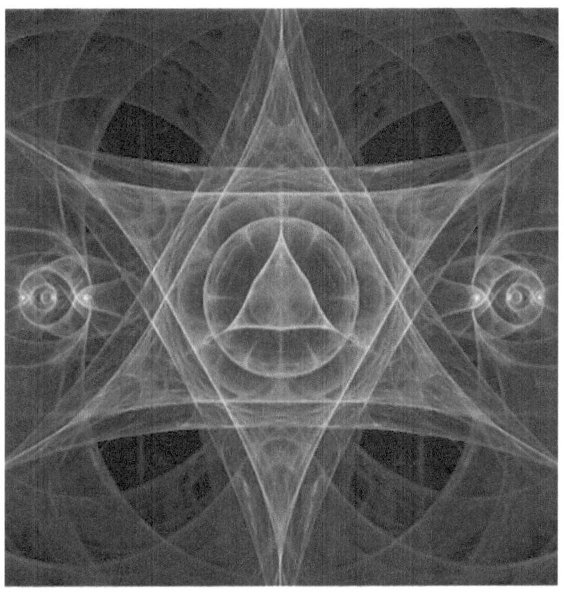

Use: To use this energy, set the intention of raising the vibration of a certain number of people, such as a neighborhood, a community, a city, or even a country! Imagine that area or group of people being enveloped in a white, shiny dome of light, and then imagine that they have increased by the level of vibration indicated. Typically, it is wise to use a percentage such as ten, or twenty percent.

Invocations that are too intense may not work or could cause an overload of energy upon those located in the area. Energy-overload symptoms include dizziness, fatigue, nausea, and a general feeling of being out of balance. This will only last a short while, one to four days; however, it is best to maintain a lower vibration increase to avoid this. All humans have free will, so it may not affect everyone however, the general rise in vibration of the area will be noticeable where the energy is being used. Use the invocation process and allow. Follow up on your work by releasing attachment to the outcome, and watch for news articles, community changes, and even city changes that indicate the area has shifted to a higher vibration

Example: I regularly received guidance to activate this energy to increase the vibration of areas of the world. Myself, and many others who are healers on this planet, may raise consciousness in this way. Any time I go into a new space I will activate the energies so that there will not be a discrepancy in energy. Empaths may find energy discrepancies to be uncomfortable and will not stay in them for long. This is also a part of the awakening of humanity and the raising of consciousness and vibration.

9

CREATION ENERGIES

These energies are more advanced, as we discussed earlier. Generally, these energies are used by healers or practitioners who are guided to do this type of work for humanity or the earth. The vibration for this work is extremely high and will only operate in the vibration of love, light, peace, unity, prosperity, and oneness in alignment with the divine God plan.

The practitioner will want to be aligned in love, light, peace, prosperity and one with God prior to using these energies. Generally, these energies work on a mass or global level, although the intention could be set only to work on a certain area of the planet. Similar to the other energies, the practitioner will set an intention for what is to be created or upgraded. Focus the energy on the intention, rather than what it is clearing or replacing. There is a method to clear that which is no longer serving us. We will discuss this shortly.

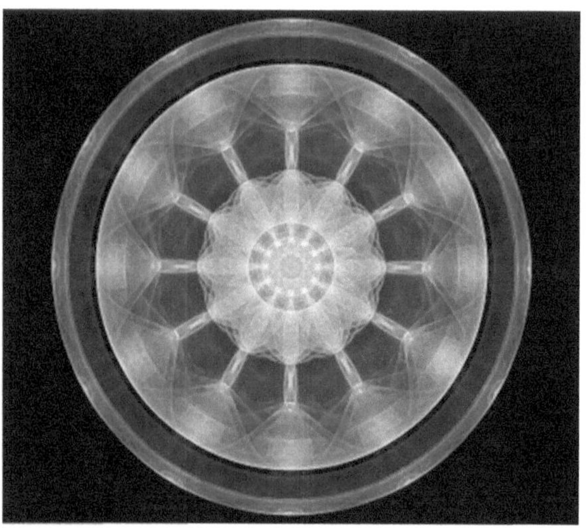

Invoking this energy while being in a pure meditative and positive state, brings about the highest results. When invoking the energy state, *"For the highest good for humanity and the mother earth and in alignment with God"* at the end of every intention. We as humans are quite smart; however, even with best intentions, we are not always aware of the highest good and diving God plan. This will allow for the energy to access the higher interdimensional levels and the angelic realms to create the highest good in a way that we cannot even perceive or fathom from our perspective here on earth.

17. ALPHAKRYON

Beginning: Use this energy for new beginnings. There are many reasons why we may want to set an intention for new beginnings. This will wipe the slate clean and make a fresh start. This can be used for mind-sets, emotional states, processes, and so many other aspects of the human existence.

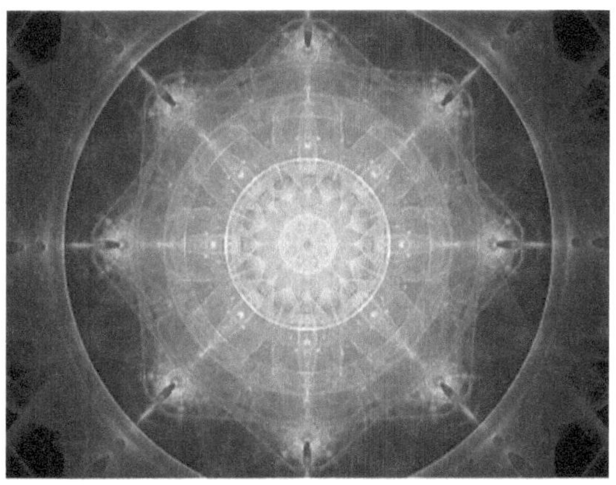

Use: For those guided to do this work, first meditate on what is being restarted and carefully prepare the intention prior to invoking this energy. Once invoked, always remember to add "for the highest good for humanity and the Mother Earth" to the intention. Focus on positive outcomes that vibrate in the higher dimensions.

Use this energy in pair with Omegakryon (ending energy) for the best results. In many cases, something must end prior to a new beginning. For instance to end poverty and begin prosperity, one would say: "Omegakryon poverty on earth, Alphakryon prosperity on earth." This is a big task in our current conditions on earth, so it may take time in the linear world for this invocation to work. It is good to do large global invocations, but also small measurable invocations will allow the healer to see more instantaneous results. In any case the results can be profound. Please note that the invocations will work when they are invoked in the highest good for humanity, earth and in alignment with the divine plan of God. Release attachments to the outcome and allow in the nonlinear fifth dimensional time free from expectations.

Example: I have used these energies for small personal healing sessions as well as global. One day I used the energies to invoke equality for women by saying: Alphakryon equality for women in all ways to men on this earth plane". I also used Omegakryon in this invocation by saying: Omegakryon all ways in which women are unequal to or treated as property of men." Within weeks there were many articles in the news about women's marches, rights movements and new rights available to women around the world. I am not giving full credit of these changes to the energies, as many of these changes have been in the plan of the universe and the collective consciousness, however I do believe the energies played a large role in amplifying the effects of the changes and empowerment. I have seen many changes occur from the invocations of the energies. This is only one example.

18. **HELIKRYON**

Sun Energy: The sun is a vital energy source for humanity. It provides light, energy, and life for earth and humanity. This energy can be used to increase the light in an area. If there are areas of darkness on earth needing energy, warmth, light, and life, this energy can be used to heal these spaces.

Use: Invoke the energy to the area needing healing and allow. Again, the timing will be according to the divine timing, rather than linear third-dimensional time.

Example: An area of the sea life and coral are dying, this energy could be invoked to this area to begin healing, and restore the natural balance of the ocean. The invocation: "Helikryon, Helikryon, Helikryon the healing of the oceans near Australia to restore life to the coral reef in the highest good for all life in that area and in alignment with the highest divine good."

19. **MENEKRYON**

Moon: The moon brings us light at night and balances many aspects of the earth. We call this the lunar cycle. Women are aligned to this cycle with their bodies and their moods, as are the oceans. When aspects of the world relate to divine feminine, nocturnal energies, or the aspects of earth regulated by the moon, this energy will be helpful in balancing these aspects.

Use: Invoke the energy using the regular process, and set the intention of which aspect of the moon needs balancing on earth. It could be that sleep cycles of humanity need to be balanced, as an example. Set the intention and say, "For the highest good of humanity and the earth." Allow the balancing to occur.

Example: Many of the hormones of women are currently out of balance due to a multitude of reasons that we will not get into. We could create an invocation such as: "Menekryon, Menekryon, Menekryon, realign the cycles and hormones of the divine feminine on earth to the natural cycles in alignment with the moon, in the highest good of women." Once we have created it, we will allow and simply watch as this evolves. These changes could occur in ways that women change the habits globally leading to the imbalances.

20. **ASTERKRYON**

Star Energy: This energy is related to the guidance of the stars. Much of our earth life is affected by the stars. There are many different beliefs and ancient texts about how the stars affect our daily lives. The Egyptians used astronomy for measurement and the creation of the pyramids. Humans throughout history have used the stars as a guidance system as well as a measurement tool. Scientists have many theories on how advanced the technology was in ancient times. My meditations and visions indicate that the technology was advanced and has been lost, as we "fell from grace" and were covered in a veil, so that humanity could find our way again. We are now at a point in time in which the veils have been lifted, and humanity is once again connected to the star energy and available to connect to the higher vibration and level of consciousness.

Use: Use this energy to connect to the stars and bring in the wisdom and the powerful energy available. This energy will be used purely by guidance through visions and meditations, as this is how the stars work. The guidance and meditations provide the intentions based on questions that are asked. Ask the question, invoke the energy, and allow the stars to guide you to set the intention needed.

21. **AETHERKRYON**

Ethers: The ethers are all which surrounds us. It is the air we breathe. From a scientific perspective it an oxygen atom connected to two alkyl or aryl groups. Our ethers can become out of balance and require balancing. There are many situations that could cause this, mostly human miscreations. When the air we breathe is out of balance or unhealthy to breathe, this energy will balance it.

Use: Use this energy for any reason that the air is not in alignment with the highest good of humanity or earth. Invoke the energy using the invocation and set the intention of the part of the air that requires balancing. Place a platinum dome over the area that is being balanced with the mind's eye and imagine the murky unhealthy air being transformed into healthy, balanced air.

Example: In a densely populated city, it may sometimes become hard to breathe when there are few trees; this energy could be used to improve the air quality of the city. When it manifests it may be found that the city plants more trees, increases public transportation or there could be a big rain that clears the air.

22. **GAMAKRYON**

Ultimate Ray: This is a ray of energy that emits large amounts of light energy. The gamma light ray is one of the strongest and most potent forms of energy available. The ray is a fine point. Unlike the other energies, which cover large spaces or are all-encompassing in an aura or an area of the earth, it can be directed to small and very specific locations like a laser. The direction can be as fine as a small needle. The thickness of the ray can vary by the intention set by the "artist." We call the practitioner an artist in this case because he or she will guide the ray mentally to create the intended "art." In Western medicine Gamma Rays are used to cure cancer and other diseases with light technology. We will use the "etheric, third eye" version.

Examples of Use: Demarcation of boundaries between areas, art and healing of the physical body. It is used in small spaces within the body for clearing out toxic energy surrounding diseased areas or cells and any way in which a pointed or fine ray may be needed. This energy generally can only be used on living cells such as plant life, animal cells, or human cells.

Use: Use the standard invocation process, set the intention, and direct the energy using the mind to the area or space where the energy is desired. For instance, if drawing a circle, use the mind's eye to direct the energy in a circle in the desired space. Results will show in divine interdimensional timing.

Example: If the kidneys of a patient are in adrenal fatigue, the practitioner could use the mind's eye to direct the ray to the kidneys. Visualize the dark area where the kidneys are underperforming and invoke the energy by saying: "Gamakryon, Gamakryon, Gamakryon clear necrosis in the kidneys and fill with the divine light of the Gama ray to heal the kidneys." Imagine the kidneys filling with the Gama Ray and healing. Allow the process to work in divine timing.

Safety: This energy must be only directed to areas where the energy is truly needed or desired by someone who has the capability to direct energy. Always ask for the highest good of the area or person where the work is being performed. We must respect the divine plan for the person we are healing. Despite family, friends wanting to save someone, the divine plan of a person will determine the ability for them to recover from a disease, and we must respect this and allow the divine plan to unfold.

23. **OMEGAKRYON**

Ending: This energy is used to complete cycles or put an end to that which no longer serves us. There are many creations on earth now. Some of them serve our highest good, and some could be recreated in an improved way that serves the higher good for humanity or earth in the higher dimensions. This energy is best used for ending what no longer serves humanity or the earth at this time. Typically, it is best to use it with **Alphakryon**, as when a cycle ends, a new cycle begins. In order to have an ending, there must be a new beginning. It is best used by those light-workers who have practice clearing earthly issues and co-creating new ones.

Use: Invoke the energy and set the intention for that which will end. Be very specific in the intention. An entire system or process does not need to end because one aspect of it no longer serves us. Identify the area or portion that no longer serves us, and set that as the intention to end. Immediately set the intention for the creation or starting of the replacement process or system using **Alphakyron**. Refer to the first energy in this section for further explanation as these two energies are often paired.

Cautions: Ensure that when the intention is set, you are not creating havoc or disruption of systems. Avoid using this energy to end livelihoods or situations that would cause undue hardship on earth or humanity. Always ask for the highest good, one with God.

Example: if the mail system we use is very slow, there is no reason to do away with the whole system. Set the intention to end the portions of the systems that are causing the slow down. An intention for this invocation could be: "Omegakryon all processes within the mail system that block the highest efficiency, Alphakryon new processes that allow mail to flow freely at the highest efficiency in the highest good for all involved and in alignment with God."

10

TWIN RAYS

Divine Feminine and Masculine Energies: These two rays are used for space preparation and healing from the perspective of balancing the divine feminine and masculine. Patricia Coates-Robles speaks of a similar set of rays in her teachings.

PLATINUM PINK RAY

The platinum ray looks exactly as it sounds, like a ray of platinum with an undertone of pink colored energy. The ray is activated using the healer's third eye or mind's eye. Use this ray to activate a specific site on earth with the divine feminine energy or within a human body. When invoked it will bring in the divine feminine energy to an area for healing.

ELECTRIC BLUE RAY

The blue ray is an electric blue color that looks similar to the electric blue color of a vibrant ocean or the Mediterranean sky. This ray is also activated from the healer's third eye or mind's eye, and is representative of the divine masculine.

Purpose: The purpose of the Twin rays is for balancing the divine feminine and masculine. The earth and humanity have been going through a process of raising in vibration, and in order to do this the divine feminine and masculine must be perfectly balanced in humans as well as earth. Earlier in the book, we discussed the **Ankryon** energy for balancing the divine feminine and masculine, we also discussed that the location for this balancing occurs in the third chakra, the seat of the soul, also known as the solar plexus. The energy of **Ankryon** may be used in combination with the Twin Rays in order to balance the feminine and masculine within a human or earthly locations. In order for our bodies and earth to increase in vibration, it is imperative that these energies be balanced regularly.

It is quite noticeable that equality of women has been increasing exponentially over the past 100 years and more and more, and the lines of roles between the sexes have blurred. The earth is going through a balancing of these energy in her own chakra system simultaneously to the human shift. The progress is tremendous.

Many spiritually awakened humans on earth have been meeting what may be termed as twin flames. These twins are typically a male and female, although sometimes same sex, that share a soul signature and are drawn together for spiritual work with what feels like a magnet.

At the beginning of this era around 2000 years ago, the whole souls split into two, which became the divine feminine and the divine masculine, in order to experience lessons in duality. We are now reaching a point in which the souls are ready to return to oneness and rebalance to become whole again. The souls may or may not incarnate at the same time, and may or may not have a physical relationship in this lifetime. They will have a similar purpose and mission on this earth and hold the same soul signature. Sometimes the same soul may incarnate in multiple bodies at the same time in the form of a soul family. The purpose of this is to learn life lessons and accomplish more in less time. Some of these souls may or may not engage in marriage or romantic relationships, but it is not necessary and often times even difficult for this type of relationship to withstand such soul level intensity. More often then not these relationships will be intense and short lived. They may also come in the form of a family member like a sister, brother or even a colleague. What is more important is the deep soul connection and vibration that they share. These meetings are important to the growth and raising of vibration of earth and humanity as these relationships are balancing these energies simply by these twins working together to resolve differences in duality. Often times the twins will have a spiritual purpose or work to do here on earth. The rays may be used to assist with these relationships. The balancing may be done on one or both of the twin flames. The balancing will occur either way.

Invocation of the Rays:

Single Ray Invocation: Imagine with the Mind's Eye that the ray is coming down from the heavens, and like a light beam is directed at the person, place or thing where the balancing is to occur.

Places: Generally the rays will work within a specific single point or location, and radiate over a larger space, which could cover several meters or miles in diameter depending on the intention set by the healer.

> ***Example:*** *If the ray were to be initiated over the peak of a mountain, it would be directed through the apex of the mountain, and the energy of the ray would radiate through the entire mountain filling the space of the mountain with the energy.*

Person: When working with a person, imagine with the mind's eye that the ray is directed to the specific area of the aura or physical body where the work is being done.

> ***Example:*** *If the heart chakra is out of balance in regards to the divine feminine, the platinum pink ray would be directed toward this chakra for healing. The healer would visualize that the chakra is filled with the ray.*

Twin Ray Invocation: Imagine that the two rays of electric blue and platinum pink are intertwined in a double helix similar to that of a DNA strand.

- **Places:** Imagine with the mind's eye that the double helix of the twin energies is directed into the area that requires the two energies to be balanced.
- **Person:** Imagine with the mind's eye that the double helix of the twin energies is aligned with the spine of the patient, starting with the bottom of the helix at the base of the sacral or first chakra and goes up to a minimum of the crown or seventh chakra, as far up to the sixteenth chakra.

Invocation Words: While imagining the helix in the space or along the spine, the following invocation will be said:

> ***"The divine feminine and divine masculine are perfectly balanced in harmony, peace, unity, oneness, prosperity in alignment with the highest divine self and the divine plan ONE with God."***

Once the invocation is complete, the balancing has occurred. This can be repeated over multiple sessions. Even with only one session, the effects will be profound.

Time: As we have mentioned throughout the book, the energies work within a non-linear time frame, so simply allow and accept the changes will occur according to divine timing.

11

∽∾

Symbols In Healing

Having lived in Egypt in the 80's I took five years of Egyptology classes during my primary studies. I now see how this was critical in my development and my understanding of this ancient technology. We may not be aware, however these symbols that we call hieroglyphs carry metaphysical energies with them. When I receive visions and guidance on how to perform healing sessions, I often see symbols as part of the work. I am going to discuss three that I use frequently.

I had the great pleasure of meeting William Henry at an Edgar Cayce and Earthkeepers conference. He writes about and photographs hieroglyphics and has excellent examples and deep discussions about the meanings of these symbols.

I use the following symbols that I combine with the Tachyon and Kryon energies. I would like to elaborate on them and share how to combine them with the energies and other healing modalities.

Ancient Egypt Symbols

Ankh

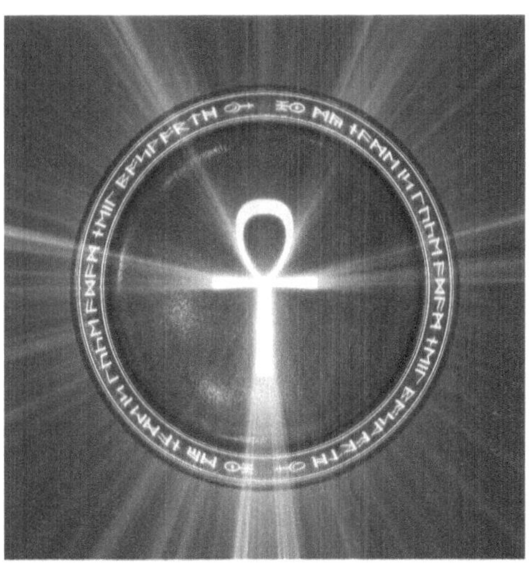

The ankh is the most important of the symbols because it indicates the key of life. I often use this in combination with the other energies as a strengthener and harmonizer. When I visualize it in the area of the healing with the energy being activated I feel a substantial increase and complete clearing occur. Visually in my mind's eye I will see energy that no longer serves dissipating instantly and allowing the energies to then bring in the balancing energies more quickly. I place the ankh on my energy centers daily and see that it quickly balances and clears my energies. Sometimes if I have had a heavy or arduous healing, I will imagine the ankh on all the energy centers and will imagine that I have released any energies I may have picked up from the client falling into a vortex below me and dissipating. I then imagine my energy body refilling with the great white light.

Crook & Flail

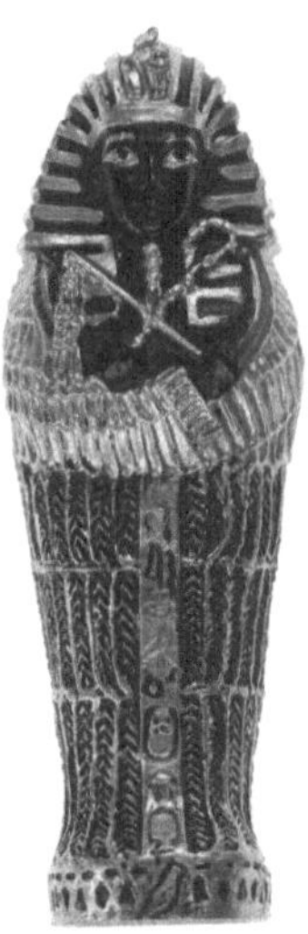

The **Crook** and the **Flail** were seen on all mummified Kings and Pharaohs in ancient Egypt. They were seen as symbols of prestige, power and protection by the ancient Egyptians. According to Bolter in the Documentary "The Pyramid Code" they also held further meaning. The crook represented the emotional body, The Flail represented the mind and the Staff represented the physical body.

I have utilized the visualization of these ancient Egyptian symbols for healing the mind, emotions and physical body in much the same way I utilized the Ankh. When activating the energies, I imagine the symbol in the area that requires healing and I imagine the healing occurring. In my case I will see shifting of energies in my mind's eye or feel a shift in the energy. When this is complete I will say "and so it is".

Scarab

This is a symbol of good luck and related to the masculine energy or the energy of the sun. I use it to bring light to an area.

Sanskrit Symbol

Ohm

Ohm symbol—I utilize this symbol when energies feel chaotic to me. This symbol is the symbol of peace in Sanskrit and holds great power for bringing peace and calming chaotic energies. I will imagine this ohm symbol over the area of the body, the space or the area of earth that is in chaos and feel that chaotic energy dissipate. I also use a vortex for the energy to dissipate into and fill the space with the appropriate great white Tachyon or Kryon energy.

About The Author

Dr. Sara Florida L.Ac, MAOM, DD, is an author, speaker, acupuncturist and integrative medicine practitioner in Texas. She specializes in mood and emotional disorders as well as digestive health. Her doctorate is in metaphysical spiritual–emotional healing. She wrote her dissertation on how the emotions lead to higher consciousness and how in turn consciousness is able to heal the emotions. Health—including mood, energy levels, and brain function—are related to the digestive function. Her treatments and therapies treat all these areas for whole-health healing. In addition to Oriental medicine, she uses yoga, meditation, and qigong therapy to help her patients with balance, injuries, pain, and mental emotional well-being.

She is an intuitive empath and uses her natural gifts in her healing. Her own journey as an empath, which caused her to be extremely sensitive to the emotions and moods in her environment, caused her to shut down emotionally as a protection mechanism, until she attended workshops in her mid-20's, that led her to understand how to work with everything she was feeling, and later heal others utilizing what she had learned. She uses the twenty four energies advanced healing technology for advanced quantum healing as a way to amplify the healing in the other modalities in her practice to release emotional blockages and disorders from all levels of the body. She does this by permission and when appropriate. Her doctoral studies are in Metaphysical Spiritual Healing from the University of Sedona. Her master's degree is in Oriental medicine from American College of Acupuncture and Oriental Medicine rated 3 nationwide and 11 globally, also considered the Harvard of OM schools. Her mentor Dr. Bing You Acupuncturist and Tai Qi master, whom she worked with for eight years, is one of the professors at this school. She did her OM Externship in two Integrated Medicine hospitals in China. She is certified in functional medicine through Go Wellness, is a Certified yoga instructor in Ashtanga yoga, which she has practiced since 2005 with Jennifer Buergurmeister. She has practiced yoga since 1994. She has been relentlessly researching emotional health, digestive health, and yoga since the 1990s at conferences and through literature as part of her own healing journey culminating into her doctorate and this book.

Healing Sessions may booked from a distance at www.24energies.com, or locally at www.healyourvibe.com

Readers of this book may receive a discounted mini intro offer for a series of three healing sessions by using code: VibeHeal

References

Bolter, Dr. Carmen. *The Pyramid Code Documentary Series 2 of 5: High Level Technology (Documentary.)*

Buna, Tibor: A64-26574 *Thermal Aspects of Long-Term Propellant Storage on the Moon.* Tibor Buna (Martin Marletta Corp., Martin Co., Baltimore Div., Propulsion and Thermodynamlcs Dept. Baltimore, Md.). (American Rocket Soclety, Annual Meeting, 17th, and Space Flight Exposition, Los Angeles, Calif., Nov. 13-18, 1962, Paper 2690-62. Journal of Spacecraft and Rockets, vol. 1, Sept.-0ct. 1964, p. 484-491. 17 refs. [For abstract see Accession no. A63-I2228 06-30]

Brainy Quotes. https://www.brainyquote.com/quotes/albert_einstein_385842 *(website)*

Cayce, Edgar. *The Power of Your Mind (Edgar Cayce Series Title).* 2010.

Cota-Robles, Patricia. *The Next Step…Re-Unification with the Presence of God Within Our Hearts.* 1989.

Cota-Robles, Patricia. *The Violet Flame: God's Gift to Humanity*. 2005.

Cross, John R. and Robert Charman. *Healing with the Chakra Energy System: Acupressure, Bodywork, and Reflexology for Total Health*. 2006.

Dale, Cyndi. *Advanced Chakra Healing*. 2005.

Dale, Cyndi. *The Subtle Body: An Encyclopedia of Your Energetic Anatomy*. 2009.

Hall, Judy. *The Art of Psychic Protection*. 2011.

Hofstadter, Douglas R. and Daniel C. Dennett. *The Mind's I: Fantasies and Reflections on Self & Soul*. 2001

Carroll, Lee. *The End Times: New Information for Personal Peace*. goodreads.com

Caroll, Lee, *Kryon.com (website)*

McLaren, Karla. *Your Aura & Your Chakras: The Owner's Manual*. 1998.

McNamara, Dr. *Joseph. https://tachyoncounseling.com/bio/.* (website)

Miller, David K. *New Spiritual Technology for the Fifth-Dimensional Earth: Arcturian Teachings from the Sacred Triangle*. 2009.

Sankey, Mikio. *Esoteric Acupuncture: Gateway to Expanded Healing, Vol. 1.* 1999.

Skinner, Stephen. *Sacred Geometry: Deciphering the Code.* 2009

Tyberonn, James. *The Alchemy of Ascension.* 2010.

Terra Tachyon. Tachyon Energy www.terratachyon.com/en/content/7-tachyon-energy

Wetzel, Lois J. *Akashic Records: Case Studies of Past Lives.* 2011.

Weissman, Dr. Darren R. *Awakening to the Secret Code of Your Mind: Your Mind's Journey to Inner Peace.* 2010.

Wojton, Djuna. *Karmic Healing: Clearing Past-Life Blocks to Present-Day Love, Health, and Happiness.* 2014.

I offer this book to healers and light workers as a gift of healing from the higher realms. May this book bring about peace, love, light, unity, oneness and prosperity in alignment with the highest divine purpose of healing humanity and earth.

~Love Dr. Sara Florida